CUMBRIA LIBRARIES

3 8003 03578 6300

Morphine and the Relief of Cancer Pain

Cumbria
County Council
Libraries, books and more . . .

1/5/09

17 AUG 10

8/19

WITHDRAWN

D0334357

Please return/renew this item by the last due date.
Library items may also be renewed by phone or
via our website.
www.cumbria.gov.uk/libraries

CLIC

Ask for a CLIC password

Beaconsfield, Bucks, UK

First edition (with Dr Sylvia Lack) published in 1987 under the title *Oral Morphine: Information for Patients, Families and Friends.* Reprinted 1988, 1990. Reprinted with revisions 1991, 1993, 1994, 1995, 1996, 1997, 1998

This edition © Robert G. Twycross 1999
Reprinted 2003, with revisions 2005

This book is copyright. All rights are reserved. Apart from any fair dealing for the purpose of private study, research, criticism or review, as permitted under the Copyright, Designs and Patents Act 1988, no part of this publication may be reproduced, stored or transmitted in any form or by any means, without the prior permission in writing of the publishers. Enquiries should be addressed to Beaconsfield Publishers at 20 Chiltern Hills Road, Beaconsfield, Bucks HP9 1PL, UK.

The author asserts his right as set out in Sections 77 and 78 of the Copyright, Designs and Patents Act 1988 to be identified as the author of this work wherever it is published commercially and whenever any adaptation of this work is published or produced including any sound recordings or films made of or based upon this work.

British Library Cataloguing in Publication Data
Twycross, Robert G.
 Morphine and the relief of cancer pain: information for
 patients, families and friends. — 2nd ed.
 1. Cancer — Palliative treatment — Popular works
 2. Cancer pain — Treatment — Popular works 3. Morphine
 I. Title II. Oral morphine 6 16.9' 94' 06 1
 ISBN 0–906584–50–7

Phototypeset by Gem Graphics, Trenance, Cornwall
in 10.75 on 12.5pt Times
Printed by Halstan & Co. Ltd, Amersham, Bucks, UK

Contents

Contents

Contents

Topic List

The numbers shown below refer to pages and not to questions

PAIN IN CANCER

Cancer is a common disorder. In developed countries, one in three people suffer from cancer at some stage in their lives. Of those who do, about one third will be completely cured; the rest have to go on living with their cancer until one day it beats them – or they die of something else.

Many patients with cancer experience pain, *but not all.* About a quarter of patients with widespread cancer never have pain. However, even if you come within the unlucky three-quarters, there is no need to suffer continuous severe pain. And for those who are dying, *a pain-free death is a realistic goal.*

In the 1980s, the World Health Organization published a book entitled *Cancer Pain Relief.* This states that:

- cancer pain can and must be treated
- drugs usually give good relief, provided the right drug is taken in the right dose at the right time intervals
- for persistent pain, the drugs should be taken regularly 'by the clock' and not 'as needed'
- the key painkillers are aspirin, codeine and morphine (or their local alternatives)
- morphine is simple to administer and achieves good pain relief in most patients when properly used, either alone or in conjunction with aspirin and other 'helper' drugs.

Of course other symptoms also need to be treated. In addition, patients and families need practical and emotional support from a doctor, a nurse or other health professional to enable them to cope with the ongoing challenge of living with cancer.

I acknowledge with gratitude the help and advice I have received over the years from my medical and nursing colleagues. In relation to this reprint, I am particularly grateful to Claire Stark-Toller.

R.T.

COMMON QUESTIONS ABOUT MORPHINE

1. What is morphine and how does it work?

Morphine is a naturally-occurring substance obtained from the opium poppy. Codeine comes from the same source. Both morphine and codeine relieve pain, cough, breathlessness and diarrhoea. Morphine is a stronger painkiller and is used mainly when codeine (or a similar drug) is not sufficient. Morphine and codeine relieve pain by blocking pain transmission in the spinal cord and brain.

2. Morphine? Does it mean I'm at the end of the road?

Many patients need morphine after a major operation, in childbirth, or after a heart attack. In these circumstances, the use of morphine clearly does *not* mean that the person is about to die. Rather, it is a help to recovery.

In cancer, morphine is used to relieve pain which does not respond to painkillers such as aspirin and codeine. It is used at many different stages of the illness, and *not* just when death is close. Some cancer patients never need morphine, though many need it for weeks or months – or occasionally for years. Others need it for just a few days.

3. Doesn't morphine speed things up – make you die sooner?

There is no evidence that this is so. Indeed, patients often take on a new lease of life when free of pain and able to sleep comfortably at night. Freed from the nightmare of never-ending pain, they gain a renewed interest in food, and in life generally.

4. Will morphine take the pain away completely?

In many cases, yes. However, relief may be incomplete with certain types of pain. For example:
- bone pain
- nerve pain
- bedsore pain.

With these pains, other drugs or treatments may be necessary in addition to, or instead of, morphine. For example, an aspirin-type of painkiller *plus* morphine is generally needed for bone pains.

Certain pains should not be treated with morphine at all, for example:

- tension headache and migraine
- muscle spasm pain
- arthritis and spondylosis.

Other remedies exist for these ailments and should be recommended by your doctor.

5. If I take morphine now, will there be anything stronger for me when the pain gets worse?

The first thing to get straight is that the pain may never get worse. If it does, an increase in the dose of morphine will control the pain again. This may be permanent, but some patients find they can reduce the dose again a few days or weeks later. This often happens, for example, after a course of radiation therapy to a painful bone.

Second, there is no need for anything stronger because the dose of morphine can be increased almost indefinitely. However, if a new pain develops which does not respond well to morphine, other treatments will need to be used.

6. Wouldn't it be better to keep off morphine until things become really unbearable?

You may be worried that your body will 'get used' to morphine and then there will be nothing left to relieve the pain. This does not happen. If a pain recurs while continuing to take morphine, it will be relieved by increasing the dose – a process which can be repeated many times if necessary.

7. Will I need bigger and bigger doses to control the pain?

Not necessarily. However, many people do need to increase the dose from time to time. On the other hand, with some people it is possible to reduce the dose, or even stop taking morphine altogether.

8. How long can I go on taking morphine? Does the effect wear off eventually?

If you need morphine you will be able to go on taking it with good effect for the rest of your life, whether this is months or years. Normally, the effect does not wear off. The common reason for an increase in the dose of morphine is that the cancer is causing more pain, not that the effect of the morphine is wearing off.

9. Will I become addicted?

What most people mean by this is, 'Will I become hooked and unable to stop the morphine, even if I no longer need it to relieve pain?' The answer is a definite No! Over several decades, I treated thousands of cancer patients with morphine but I never had difficulty stopping treatment because of addiction.

On the other hand, it is unwise to stop long-term morphine therapy abruptly. If you no longer need morphine, the dose is best reduced step by step under your doctor's supervision. Thus, after radiation therapy for bone pain, for example, the dose of morphine can be reduced progressively over two to three weeks.

The reason for a gradual dose reduction is because most people who take morphine regularly for several weeks or months develop 'physical dependence'. This is not the same as addiction. It means that if morphine is stopped suddenly and completely, you would experience withdrawal symptoms, for example feel unwell generally and have diarrhoea.

The dose of morphine needed to prevent withdrawal symptoms is only about a quarter of the previously used pain-relieving dose. Thus, after a successful injection to deaden a painful nerve (a 'nerve block'), it is possible immediately to halve the dose of morphine (or even more) – and to continue reducing the dose more slowly after that – without any upset at all.

STARTING TREATMENT WITH MORPHINE

10. Now that I'm starting morphine, what are the important things I need to know about it?

- For most people, the best way to take morphine is by mouth
- solutions and short-acting tablets should be taken regularly every 4 hours
- most types of long-acting tablets provide relief for 12 hours, and a few for 24 hours; but in practice some patients take long-acting tablets every 8 hours
- the dose needs to be adjusted to meet your personal requirements
- the main unwanted effects are vomiting and constipation; these can be treated effectively (see Questions 26 and 32)
- you may need other drugs and treatments as well as morphine
- your response to morphine must be carefully monitored, particularly during the first few days and weeks.

11. What's the difference between morphine in solution ('liquid morphine') and morphine tablets?

Morphine works equally well whether given in solution or as tablets. However, morphine solutions have a bitter taste, which many patients dislike. Some commercial preparations have a masking flavour, others don't. To improve palatability, consider adding a flavour of your choice (fruit juice, milk, etc.) after you have poured the liquid morphine into the medicine cup. There is a long-acting morphine suspension – supplied as granules to be mixed with water. Although tasteless, the suspension is not widely used because it is much more expensive.

Tablets come in two varieties and several different brands: short-acting ('immediate release') and long-acting ('sustained release'). Most patients start either on morphine solution or short-acting tablets every 4 hours. Once the dose is stable, most people prefer long-acting tablets because they need to be taken only once or twice a day. The most commonly used long-acting tablets are the twice-a-day kind ('every 12 hours'), taken after breakfast and bedtime or, if easier, at 8 a.m. and 8 p.m. Although manufacturers encourage 'brand loyalty', there is no firm evidence that switching brands causes problems.

12. How do you decide how much morphine I need?

Most patients starting morphine regularly by mouth have previously been taking codeine (or a similar drug), and will start on morphine 5–10 mg every 4 hours. On the other hand, if you have been on an alternative to morphine, the starting dose will be higher, perhaps 30 mg or even 60–100 mg every 4 hours.

13. What if the starting dose does not completely relieve my pain?

In case the starting dose is inadequate, you will be advised to take an extra dose after, say, 1–2 hours and again as necessary until the pain eases. The aim will be to increase the regular dose step by step until the pain is fully relieved, using rescue doses as necessary for 'topping up' during the process of 'dose titration'. You will be guided in this by your doctor or nurse.

14. Why every four hours? Wouldn't it make more sense if I just took the morphine when the pain comes back?

Actually, no. As in many other situations, anticipation is the best policy. Think for a moment of people with diabetes: they don't wait until they feel unwell before they take their next dose of insulin. Instead, with the help of a doctor or nurse, they work out how much insulin they need to keep the body sugar levels in balance and inject this regularly once or twice a day. In this way they *prevent* things from getting out of control. This is what we aim to do when treating your pain with morphine.

Think for a moment about your situation: you know from hard experience that your pain will come back when the effect of the morphine wears off. So if you take morphine 'as needed', you will be prescribing for yourself alternating periods of comfort and pain – because the pain has to return before the next dose is taken. The next dose will probably take 30–40 minutes to ease the pain again, so this would mean perhaps one hour of pain five to six times each 24 hours. Given this is avoidable pain, it is crazy to handle things that way. With morphine solutions and short-acting tablets, *regularly every four hours* is the recipe for the best combination of good round-the-clock pain relief and the least possible unwanted effects. On the other hand, very old patients (85+) and those with poorly functioning kidneys will probably be all right if they take it less often, say every 6 hours.

15. What should I do if the pain returns before the next regular dose is due?

When you start treatment with morphine, you should be told what to do if you get an unexpected return of pain ('breakthrough pain') or if you get pain repeatedly towards the end of the period between regular doses ('end-of-dose pain').

Generally, with breakthrough pain, you should take an *extra* ('rescue') dose of morphine; either half or the same as your regular every 4 hours dose. (Your doctor will advise you which is more appropriate for you.) If you are taking long-acting morphine tablets, you will need to use short-acting morphine tablets or solution in this situation. In this case, the rescue dose will be one-fifth to one-third of your 12-hourly dose, rounded up or down to a convenient number of tablets or millilitres.

With recurring end-of-dose pain, the right course of action is to increase the regular dose – although in the short term you may need to take a rescue dose as for breakthrough pain. Only rarely is it right to decrease the dose intervals to every 3 hours (ordinary tablets) or every 8 hours (long-acting tablets). So, if there is recurring end-of-dose pain, you should discuss it with your doctor who will give you the correct advice for your individual circumstances and needs.

16. What should I do if I get behind with my medication?

In hospital, it should be possible to be fairly precise about 'every 4 hours' (2 a.m., 6 a.m., 10 a.m., 2 p.m., 6 p.m. and 10 p.m.), though nursing restrictions may make the ideal difficult to achieve. In practice, most patients do not wake up on the dot of 6 a.m. In consequence, we recommend that 6 a.m. is taken to mean 'on waking'. This means that the 6 a.m. dose might not be taken until 6.30, 7 a.m., and sometimes later. Even so, the next dose should be taken at 10 a.m., and then by the clock for the rest of the day. In other words, *if you get behind, catch up at the next dose.* If you delay, you may find you have difficulty remembering a different time schedule every day. 'On waking, 10 a.m., 2 p.m., 6 p.m.' is easy to handle because it is easy to remember.

At 10 p.m. the same flexibility should be allowed as at 6 a.m. Because some people like to go to bed at, say, 9 p.m. (and are fast asleep by

10 p.m.), it is best for most patients to regard 10 p.m. and 'at bedtime' as interchangeable. If your day does not start till 9 a.m. and you never go to bed until midnight, a more individual timetable may be necessary – but the principle of every four hours by the clock remains the same.

17. How soon will I become pain-free?

This depends on your individual circumstances. Some benefit is generally seen immediately. However, if you have several pains, or if you are depressed or anxious, it could take two to three weeks to achieve maximum relief.

The first goal is to get you a good night's sleep and to make you more comfortable during the day. The second goal is complete relief at rest during the day. The final goal is freedom from pain when walking and doing things. This third level of relief is not always possible with drugs alone. In fact, some people need to limit certain activities if they continue to cause pain.

18. What about the nights? Do I need to set my alarm clock for 2 a.m.?

In theory, yes but, in practice, almost always no. If you are elderly and in the habit of waking in the early hours to empty your bladder, a 2 a.m. dose can easily be included. In this case, after you take your bedtime dose, put out the 2 a.m. dose beside the bed for when you wake. This prevents you having to fumble around sorting out the right dose when it is dark and possibly when only half awake.

If you wake again later in the night, the empty medicine cup will indicate that you have had your 2 a.m. dose. There will be no need to rack your brain trying to remember whether you've taken it. As with 6 a.m. and 10 p.m., you can be flexible. If you wake to empty your bladder at 1 a.m. – take the 2 a.m. medicine then. If you wake free of pain at 3 a.m. – take it then.

On the other hand, if you do not regularly wake to empty your bladder during the night, there is probably no need to take a 2 a.m. dose; the reason for this is explained in the next section.

19. I've been advised to take a double dose at bedtime. Won't that be dangerous?

Most patients get through the night without a 2 a.m. dose provided they take a double dose at bedtime. A double dose increases the amount of morphine in your body, and this will cause drowsiness. Although this would be a disadvantage during the day, it is clearly an advantage at night. By the morning, the amount of morphine in your body will be back to usual levels before the first daytime dose.

We have information on file which confirms that a double dose at bedtime is definitely no more dangerous than a single dose at 10 p.m. and another one at 2 a.m. For most patients, therefore, 'every four hours' means 'on waking, 10 a.m., 2 p.m., 6 p.m., and a double dose at bedtime'.

20. Why do I have to take it so often? Couldn't I have a stronger tablet and take it less often?

With short-acting morphine tablets, 'every 4 hours' gives the best combination of maximum pain relief and minimum unwanted effects. Long-acting tablets are available for patients on a stable dose, to be taken either every 12 hours or every 24 hours depending on the make.

21. What will happen to me if morphine doesn't relieve my pain?

For many pains it is necessary to combine morphine with an aspirin-type drug to obtain satisfactory relief. The combination is particularly effective in bone pain. Morphine blocks pain transmission mainly in the spinal cord and brain, whereas aspirin-type drugs act mainly at the site of the pain.

For nerve pain, a cortisone-like drug and other 'helper' drugs are often prescribed. The commonly used 'helper' drugs for nerve pain are marketed as antidepressants and anti-epileptics – however, in this situation, they act as painkillers by enhancing the mechanisms which block pain transmission in the spinal cord.

Pain treatment also includes many non-drug measures, for example:

- psychological support for you and your family
- relaxation therapy, massage, and acupuncture
- radiation therapy (particularly for bone pain)
- injections to deaden nerves (used occasionally)
- limiting certain activities if they make the pain worse.

22. Does it matter when I take the morphine in relation to meals?

No. The times when people eat vary; it is not necessary to take this into account when taking oral morphine.

23. Can I have alcoholic drinks while taking morphine?

Bottles containing morphine tablets or solution often have a 'Do not take alcohol' label on them. This is standard cautionary advice. However, it is an oversimplification – and unnecessarily restrictive. Morphine can cause drowsiness, and this can be made worse by alcohol. So, a sensible guideline is: *while on morphine halve the amount of alcohol you consume.*

So, half a pint of beer instead of a full pint or one glass of wine instead of two, etc. More important, of course, is the *absolute* prohibition on alcohol if you plan to drive while on morphine – until the car is safely locked away for the rest of the day (see Question 24).

24. Can I drive my car while I'm taking morphine?

Doctors have a legal responsibility to advise patients if a disability is likely to make them a danger when driving. In many countries, there is an obligation on the driver to report any such disability to the licensing authority, unless relatively short-term (for example, less than three months).

Taking morphine for medicinal reasons does *not* automatically disqualify you from driving. However, your general alertness and reaction time may be affected.

It is important that you take the following precautions, particularly if you have not driven for some weeks because of ill health:

- don't drive in the dark or when conditions are bad
- don't drink alcohol, however little, during the day
- check your fitness to drive in the following way:
  choose a quiet time of the day when the light is good choose an area where there are quiet roads
  take a companion (for example husband, wife, friend)
  drive for 10–15 minutes on quiet roads
- if both you and your companion are happy with your alertness, concentration, reactions and general ability, then it's all right to drive for short distances
- don't exhaust yourself by long journeys.

Many patients receiving morphine are not well enough to drive and have no wish to do so. To drive or not to drive is therefore an issue only for a minority.

WORKING THROUGH ANY UNWANTED EFFECTS

25. Doesn't morphine have a lot of unwanted effects?

The common unwanted effects seen with morphine are:

When starting treatment	*Continuing*
nausea	constipation
drowsiness	
unsteadiness	*Occasional*
confusion	dry mouth
	sweating

Although this may seem a disturbing list, it is in fact uncommon for oral morphine to be abandoned because of unwanted effects. Early unwanted effects generally diminish with time. These issues are discussed further in the following sections. *Note that addiction is not listed.*

26. Will I need medication to counteract nausea and vomiting?

If you vomit soon after taking morphine, it will not be absorbed, the pain will continue, and you will lose confidence in its effectiveness. To avoid this, some doctors recommend the routine use of an anti-vomiting drug when morphine is prescribed. Others prescribe for selected patients only.

You will certainly need to take an antivomiting drug if:

- you are already troubled by nausea and vomiting
- you have vomited while taking codeine or one of its alternatives
- you have vomited with morphine or similar drugs in the past.

You probably will *not* need an antivomiting drug if:

- you have no nausea and vomiting at present
- you have already taken codeine or another morphine-like drug regularly without nausea and vomiting.

27. Will I have to go on taking antivomiting drugs?

Vomiting with morphine is sometimes just an initial effect. Your doctor may, therefore, reduce the dose of the antivomiting drug or phase it out altogether after you have been on a stable dose of morphine for one to two weeks. If you then feel nauseated or the vomiting recurs, this indicates that you need to stay on an antivomiting drug.

28. Will I get drowsy on morphine?

Like vomiting, drowsiness may occur during the first few days, possibly up to a week. It may recur if the dose of morphine is increased. You should persevere in the knowledge that it will get less after a few days.

Occasionally, particularly in the very old and frail, it is necessary to reduce the dose of morphine and then increase it again more slowly, every two to three days, until adequate relief is obtained.

29. Will I go on feeling drowsy and drugged?

Occasionally, yes. It is important to distinguish between persistent drowsiness and inactivity drowsiness. Most patients receiving morphine 'catnap' with ease, i.e. you may drop off to sleep if sitting quietly and alone. This can be an advantage if you have limited energy and require more sleep than you did before you developed cancer. On the other hand, if your energy is not too limited, you will be able to live a relatively normal life.

If you continue to feel drugged, and find that you can't concentrate for long and are always falling asleep, your doctor may suggest changing to an alternative morphine-like drug. However, other causes of drowsiness should first be excluded by your doctor – particularly tranquillisers and certain sleeping tablets.

30. Will morphine make me confused? Will I be safe on my own?

If you are elderly, you may become muddled at times during the first few days of treatment with morphine, but persevere – your mind will clear. If you live alone, your doctor will probably start you on a lower dose than usual if he or she thinks confusion is likely. If you (or your doctor) are worried by this possibility, it may be necessary to arrange an inpatient admission for four or five days while the morphine is started; it is however unusual to need to do this. A few patients taking morphine experience hallucinations or have other disturbing psychological effects. Such feelings may pass off spontaneously or settle with suitable additional medication.

31. Will morphine make me dizzy?

If you are elderly, you may experience dizziness or feel unsteady for a few days. However, you should continue with the morphine because this unpleasant sensation will decrease as your body adjusts to the morphine. For some people the problem occurs either just early morning or when standing up. In this case, get into the habit of pausing for several seconds when you stand up and hold on to a piece of furniture until you feel steady.

32. Will morphine make me constipated?

Yes, almost certainly you will become constipated. For most people, this is the most troublesome unwanted effect of morphine treatment. You should seek advice from your doctor about laxatives, and together learn to manage your bowels effectively.

Normally your doctor will prescribe a laxative when morphine is started. The following should be noted:

- the dose of laxative varies from person to person
- the dose may need to be adjusted several times to get it right for you
- if the laxatives don't seem to be working, seek advice sooner rather than later
- aim for a bowel movement every second or third day; more often is a bonus
- if you have no bowel movement for three days, use a laxative suppository or arrange for an enema to be given by a nurse
- drink plenty of fluids
- prune juice in the mornings can help
- adding fibre to your diet is generally not effective in counteracting constipation caused by morphine and other painkillers.

33. Since starting morphine tablets, my mouth has been very dry. What can I do about this?

You are quite right to blame the morphine, although for most people it is not a problem. However, sometimes it's a second drug you're taking which is the main culprit – and it may be possible to reduce or change that. If caused just by the morphine, you will need to moisten the mouth regularly – possibly with sips of ice-cold water or carbonated mineral water.

Other tips include increasing the flow of saliva by sucking a solid object or something acid – acid-drops cover both options and can be very helpful if you like them. Some people suck pineapple chunks or ice chips.

34. I've been sweating a lot since I started the morphine. Is this connected?

Yes, it may well be. The sweating can be heavy and is often more marked at night. Try to lower the room temperature and sleep in thin cotton nightclothes, with a change of nightclothes nearby in case the sweating is severe. Sometimes, paracetamol, an aspirin-like drug or an anti-secretory drug may be helpful If a problem, you should discuss this with your doctor.

35. What happens if I can't tolerate morphine?

In some patients, morphine slows down stomach emptying so much that they feel nauseated and vomit, despite the fact that they have been prescribed an antivomiting drug. In this case, it will be necessary to change to a drug which speeds up stomach emptying. If this doesn't sort the problem out, it may be necessary to change to an alternative painkiller.

Occasionally a patient complains of itching with morphine. If this happens with you, your doctor may recommend a change from morphine to an alternative painkiller. However, this is not often necessary; oral morphine has an excellent track record when used carefully under supervision.

36. What are the alternatives to morphine? Will they be as effective in controlling my pain?

There are several alternatives to morphine, often collectively called 'strong opioids'. Their availability varies from country to country. Buprenorphine, fentanyl, hydromorphone, methadone and oxycodone are all used at times. Diamorphine, a modified form of morphine available only in the UK, is much more soluble than morphine. This means that the volume of an injection can be smaller; it is therefore generally used when injections are necessary in the UK.

The features which may make an alternative strong opioid preferable are:

- buprenorphine is a sublingual (under-the-tongue) tablet, and therefore does not need to be swallowed; also available as a skin patch which is changed every three days
- fentanyl is administered as a skin patch, and likewise is replaced every three days
- hydromorphone and oxycodone are sometimes better tolerated than morphine, and can be tried if morphine continues to cause major unwanted effects
- methadone is useful for the few patients in whom increasing doses of morphine yields little or no benefit.

Generally, all strong opioids are as effective as morphine in controlling pain. However, buprenorphine has a ceiling dose above which one of the other strong opioids would need to be substituted. Methadone has a dual mechanism of action and, when used in cases of 'morphine failure', it is sometimes much more effective than morphine. However, it is a harder drug to use than morphine, and is therefore generally reserved for specialist use.

STILL MORE QUESTIONS ABOUT MORPHINE

37. I have excellent relief with the present dose of morphine, but once or twice a week the pain recurs. Is there anything I can do about this?

Occasional breakthrough pain is experienced by many patients. It may relate to increased activity or tiredness, or may come completely 'out of the blue'. If you experience breakthrough pain, an extra dose of short-acting morphine should be taken (see Question 15). Because an immediate effect is needed, long-acting tablets are not suitable.

If pain recurs between most or all regular doses, it probably means that the regular dose needs to be increased. Seek direction from your doctor or nurse about this. Keeping a record of when you need the extra doses can help your doctor decide on the best course of action.

38. My hands are shaky and it's difficult to handle tablets and liquid medication. What's the best way for me to take morphine?

The best option is probably to use a skin patch containing fentanyl or buprenorphine. However, with fentanyl, for rescue medication, you would still need to use morphine. Your doctor can prescribe plastic 'unit dose vials' (see Question 39), or your pharmacist can fill up some syringes with the correct amount of morphine in them for use if needed. Squirting morphine into your mouth from a unit dose vial or syringe is generally possible, even with shaky hands.

39. I'm going on holiday shortly. What's the best way of taking liquid morphine when on public transport?

For patients using liquid morphine every 4 hours and who have to travel, it is possible to obtain supplies of morphine in the plastic unit dose vials just mentioned. The top is twisted off and the contents squirted into the mouth by squeezing the vial. Several strengths are available (10 mg, 30 mg and 100 mg) and, by combining vials of different strengths, it is possible to give a range of doses in this way.

40. My problem is shortness of breath, not pain; so why have I been put on morphine?

If your breathing has become very rapid because of cancer affecting the lungs, morphine helps by slowing down the rate of breathing. As a result you will feel more comfortable and are less likely to end up gasping for breath when you do things. Many of the extra breaths you take are not really necessary and rapid shallow breathing is inefficient; slower deeper breaths are much more beneficial.

The dose of morphine to relieve breathlessness is generally smaller than doses used to relieve pain. However, as always, the benefits must be weighed against any unwanted effects. The aim of the morphine is to make you less short of breath and more relaxed. But, as with pain, morphine is not always the whole answer. If the breathlessness relates to a second disorder such as asthma, bronchitis or heart failure, treatments other than morphine will be necessary – although in severe heart failure morphine is helpful alongside other treatments.

41. Is oral morphine effective? Aren't injections better?

It is only rarely necessary to prescribe morphine by injection because oral morphine is not working. Oral morphine achieves a more constant drug level in the body, resulting in good pain relief and fewer unwanted effects. Injections tie you to a second person unless you are able to give your own. On the other hand, if you need injections because you can't swallow easily or tend to vomit up your medication, then injections make sense.

Nowadays repeated injections have been largely replaced by a gadget called a 'syringe driver'. The commonly used varieties in the UK are battery-driven and are worn in a holster. The contents of the syringe are injected just under the skin through an indwelling needle ('butterfly needle'), generally over 24 hours. At home, the syringe is normally refilled by a district nurse, though some patients and families undertake this task themselves.

42. Is it necessary to give more morphine by mouth than by injection?

Yes. As a general rule, the dose of morphine should be doubled when changing from injections to tablets or an oral solution. This is because some of the morphine is inactivated by the liver before it reaches the spinal cord and brain. Occasionally it is necessary to increase to three times the previously injected dose.

43. Are morphine injections ever needed?

Yes. Injections are necessary if you are:

- vomiting a lot
- unable to swallow.

Once the vomiting has been controlled using an antivomiting drug (also given by injection), it is often possible to change back to medicines by mouth. Nowadays, the likelihood is that a syringe driver will be used rather than injections every four hours.

44. What about 'spinal' morphine?

Spinal morphine is used, often with a local anaesthetic, in several situations – in childbirth and after some major operations, for example. In cancer, spinal morphine is used in less than 5% of patients when oral morphine together with other drugs are not effective. Most commonly this is with some nerve pains. By depositing morphine close to the spinal cord, it is possible to get a very high concentration locally where it is needed without excessive amounts elsewhere causing unwanted effects. Spinal morphine is generally administered via a syringe driver or by a small reservoir implanted below the skin.

45. Once on injections, is it possible to change successfully to the oral route?

Yes, but it may be wise to convert to the oral route in stages. For example, the antivomiting drug can be changed first, followed the next day by the morphine. The 'run-in' period with the other medication gives guidance as to whether oral administration is going to be successful. A step-by-step conversion may also be necessary if you find it difficult to believe that oral medication will be effective.

46. Can morphine be given by suppository?

Yes. Morphine suppositories are available in a range of strengths, and can also be made locally by a pharmacist. The same amount is given by suppository as by mouth. Suppositories are a useful alternative, particularly at home, if swallowing suddenly becomes impossible. If necessary, they can also be inserted into a colostomy.

47. Why do some people need more morphine than others?

There are many reasons why, including:
- differences in the severity of pain
- individual differences in sensitivity to pain
- the cause of the pain – some pains are poorly-responsive to morphine
- differences in how the body inactivates morphine
- whether other painkillers and non-drug treatments are being used
- the presence or absence of other symptoms.

48. Why do they create such a fuss about morphine in hospital? If there is only one registered nurse on duty, I often have to wait ages until one comes from the next ward.

The fuss relates to legal requirements. Certain drugs, morphine included, are 'scheduled' or 'controlled'. This means double-checking and careful book-keeping – hence the second nurse. The regulations are to prevent drugs which are attractive to addicts from getting into the wrong hands. The regulations are *not* intended to prevent cancer patients from receiving an adequate amount of morphine. It is upsetting if a shortage of nurses has this effect.

49. I've been prescribed morphine but my son who lives at home with me is a registered drug addict. How can I be sure he won't misuse my medication?

Unfortunately, you can't be sure that he won't misuse your medication, but this is unlikely if he is receiving 'maintenance' supplies of morphine or methadone for himself from an official source. However, as always, it is important not to put temptation in a person's way, so the least you should do is to keep your tablets locked away. Also, make a note of how many tablets you have in each new bottle and keep that record somewhere safe. Then if the number of tablets decreases at too fast a rate, you will know that someone – presumably your son – is helping himself. Another option, which would reduce the number of morphine tablets kept at home, would be to use buprenorphine or fentanyl skin patches.

QUESTIONS FROM A RELATIVE OR CLOSE FRIEND

50. I don't want him to know he's on morphine. Will it say on the bottle that it's morphine?

The bottle may be clearly labelled 'morphine', or it may simply be called by the brand name. However, there is no good reason for secrecy, and it should be discouraged. The reason why some families prefer secrecy is fear – based on false ideas of what morphine is and does.

Of course people may receive a mental jolt when they learn that morphine is being prescribed. It seems to indicate that things are much more serious. However, a few days later most patients are pleased to be taking it – because of greatly improved comfort. Because they are more comfortable and sleeping better, they have renewed interest in life. These and other positives generally outweigh any negatives.

21

Some patients need morphine, either continuously or periodically, for several months or even years. To commence morphine does not necessarily mean someone is close to death. Rather, it means that the patient has a severe pain that requires something stronger than codeine.

51. Is it necessary to keep the morphine locked up?

It is very rare for patients to have an oral solution of morphine stolen by members of the family or friends. However, as with all medicines, it is advisable to keep morphine out of sight in a cupboard where young children cannot reach it.

52. Is it all right to keep the bottle of morphine with the other medicines?

Yes. Most morphine solutions have a preservative in them to prevent fungi and yeasts from growing in them. However, in very hot weather it may be best to keep the morphine in a refrigerator.

53. When should morphine be taken in relation to other medicines?

It is generally best to link all the patient's medicines to the times that the morphine is taken. Thus a heart tablet taken once a day can be linked to either 6 a.m. or 10 a.m. Laxatives, too, can often be linked to the bedtime morphine. Other tablets may be linked to 10 a.m. and bedtime, or 10 a.m., 2 p.m., and 6 p.m. This will depend on how many times a day the tablets have to be taken, and whether they have to be spaced out around the clock.

54. Will the morphine mix all right with his other medicines?

Occasionally, because morphine delays stomach emptying in some patients, the combination of morphine and, for example, a cortisone-like drug may result in acid indigestion, whereas either alone would not. Similarly, the combined use of morphine and certain tranquillisers may together cause drowsiness, whereas either alone does not.

Provided the doctor is alert to such possibilities, the necessary corrective action can be taken. Generally, however, morphine can be taken at the same time as all other medication.

55. Since he has had the pain his appetite has gone completely. Will the morphine help him to eat better?

Many people lose interest in eating, and in life generally, if their whole horizon becomes one of severe never-ending pain. This is particularly so if sleep has been disturbed and the patient is exhausted both physically and mentally. In these circumstances, better pain relief and adequate sleep are likely to result in an improved appetite.

There are many reasons for loss of appetite in cancer. This means that, if the patient continues to be uninterested in food despite good pain relief, the doctor will need to assess the problem separately.

56. He's a heavy smoker and can't give up. Will this affect the dose of morphine he'll need to take?

Although smoking is generally to be discouraged, this is one situation where it would be unreasonable to make the patient feel guilty about not being able to kick the habit. Fortunately, smoking has no effect on the way in which the body handles morphine – it will be just as effective whether or not he continues to smoke.

57. Will she be safe looking after the baby if she is taking morphine?

Breast-feeding is not advisable if the mother is taking morphine because some of the morphine will be transferred to the child in the mother's milk. This question however usually refers to a toddler rather than a baby, and the answer depends more on the mother's general stamina than anything else. Most mothers in this position find the incessant demands of a pre-school child impossible to cope with and some kind of child-minding has to be arranged.

In short, provided she has enough energy, there is no reason why a mother taking morphine should be discouraged from caring for her child. Indeed, because she will be more comfortable, being on morphine is likely to enable a young mother to cope better than would otherwise be the case.

58. She's partially sighted, fiercely independent, and lives alone. Does this rule out oral morphine for her?

No, not at all. There are several different types of plastic box available from pharmacies divided into days and times. The various tablets and capsules are put into the appropriate compartments ahead of time by the pharmacist, district nurse or a relative. All the patient has to do is to tip out the contents of the next compartment at the right time – and swallow them! This gets round the need to open several bottles of tablets when medication is due, and greatly reduces the likelihood of a mistake through opening the wrong bottles.

Further, by converting to a once-a-day long-acting preparation of morphine, most medication could be given just once a day with the help of a relative, friend or district nurse. Another option is to use a fentanyl or buprenorphine skin patch. Each patch lasts for three days and, if necessary, could be changed by a district nurse.

59. What about signing legal documents while taking morphine?

It all depends on the patient's general circumstances. For most patients, the use of morphine brings about an improvement in their general condition. However, if someone becomes very drowsy or muddled when starting morphine, it would be best to delay signing important documents for a few days. This will make it difficult at a later date for another person to cast doubt on the patient's mental state at the time of signing.

60. What should I do if he insists on having more morphine than he's been prescribed? Could it kill him?

If left to their own devices, patients are more likely to take too little rather than too much. Assuming that the desire for more morphine is to relieve distressing pain, there are no grounds for refusing the request. If more than a double or treble dose is insisted on, there may have to be a certain resistance:

'I'll give you a double dose now, and then ring Dr X. to let him know the prescribed dose is not holding the pain. If he says to give more, that's fine. I just think we need guidance.'

Should the patient receive too much, it will most probably act like the bedtime double dose (see Question 19). The patient will sleep for several hours and wake refreshed and free of pain.

61. Is there a danger that she'll use the morphine to commit suicide?

Some cancer patients, if caught up in a living hell of unrelieved pain, think of killing themselves. Surprisingly few do. In my experience, when the pain is relieved – often with morphine – the patient no longer thinks of suicide. Out of several thousand cancer patients I have cared for, none has used morphine to commit suicide.

62. If he has no pain and refuses to take the next dose, do I insist on him taking it?

It depends on the circumstances. If the patient is confused, the refusal may be unreasonable, and continued pressure to accept the morphine may be necessary. On the other hand, if the confusion is associated with paranoia (feelings of being threatened or persecuted), even gentle persuasion might make matters worse. If in doubt, seek help from a doctor or nurse, possibly by phone in the first instance.

If not confused, he will presumably have a rational reason for declining the morphine. Possibly it is causing unacceptable drowsiness, or intolerable nausea, or severe unrelieved constipation is felt to be worse than the cancer pain. There is clearly a need to explore the reasons behind the refusal.

63. If she becomes unconscious, should the morphine be discontinued?

Even if the patient is unconscious and death is expected within hours or days, it is important to continue giving morphine (generally by injection). This is for two reasons:

- unconscious patients in pain become restless
- 'physical dependence' generally develops after several weeks of treatment with morphine.

If physical dependence has developed, and the morphine is stopped abruptly, the patient will become restless. If the degree of physical dependence is considerable, she might also sweat a lot and develop severe diarrhoea and be incontinent.

On the other hand, if the patient becomes unconscious unexpectedly, you should seek help from a nurse or doctor. They will advise you on the best course of action after re-assessing the situation. In this circumstance, it may well be appropriate to omit or reduce the next dose.

FINAL THOUGHTS

Pain is not a simple sensation like seeing or hearing: it is much more complex. Four thousand years ago, Aristotle described pain as 'a passion of the soul' – a poetic way of emphasizing that pain represents a major area of body-mind interaction. Intensity of pain is modified not only by medication but also by the person's mood and morale, and the meaning of the pain for that person. Living with cancer is hard work and there are often plenty of negative factors to contend with – loss of energy, loss of job, loss of financial independence and so on. All these factors, and more, influence how sensitive we are to any underlying physical pain signals.

The diagram below shows why companionship and the support of family and friends are so important. Equally important is the support of an attentive doctor and nurse; they are just as necessary as the right medication. The two work together; either alone is not enough.

Other symptoms
Adverse effects of treatment
Insomnia and chronic fatigue

PHYSICAL

PSYCHOLOGICAL		SOCIAL
Anger at delays in diagnosis		Worry about family and finances
Anger at therapeutic failure	**TOTAL**	Loss of job prestige and income
Disfigurement	**PAIN**	Loss of social position
Fear of pain and/or death		Loss of role in family
Feelings of helplessness		Feelings of abandonment and isolation

SPIRITUAL
Why has this happened to me?
Why does God allow me to suffer like this?
What's the point of it all?
Is there any meaning or purpose in life?
Can I be forgiven for past wrongdoing?